# PROSTATE CANCER
# THE RACE
# TO
# FINISH LAST!

## RAFIQ BANDUKWALA

With my own decade-long Prostate Cancer Journey, I have written this book for thousands of men, <u>WITH LIMITED MEDICAL KNOW-HOW</u>, to understand the Six Supporting Pillars, to better navigate their own **PROSTATE CANCER JOURNEY!**

Copyright @ 2024 by Rafiq Bandukwala LLC. All rights reserved. Printed in the United States of America. No part of this book may be used reproduced whatsoever without written permission except in the case of brief questions embodied in critical articles or reviews.

Second Edition 2024

# DEDICATION

To my family and friends
and especially
to my companion and best friend of
over 50 years
my wife Lalita
and
for having made life a very pleasant journey
to
Ibrez, Claire, Aydin, Laith,
Shaheen, Nick, Zayn and Xavier!

# ACKNOWLEDGEMENTS

To the Oncology team (headed by the brilliant and compassionate Dr. Daniel George and his very proficient team of prostate cancer specialist physicians, radiation oncologists, medical oncologists, physician assistants, research nurses, dieticians) at Duke Cancer Center, Durham, North Carolina, USA, who have given me guidance and treatments and support on my prostate cancer journey over the past decade.

Special acknowledgement to Dr. Daniel George, who with my previous writing experience of the book titled DON'T RE'TIRE', RE'FRESH'! A Refreshing Look at Retirement! (available on Amazon), motivated me to write this book and together came up with the title of this book.

Special acknowledgement also to my personable and talented Urologist, Dr. Robert Medairos of Duke Clinic, Durham, North Carolina.

To my family and friends, who over the years, have brought me many, many smiles and especially have been my mental, physical and emotional support over the past decade on my prostate cancer journey.

A very special thank you to Anita and Mike Misko, Debbie Marshall, Jodi Taylor, Anissa Clark, Kathleen Privette, Kaija LaValle, Kathy Mulligan, Statira Sirur, Darshana and Bankim Wani, Maria Marty, Colleen Miller, Julie Tisdale, Janet Marshall, Julie Overby and more for their caring and their unconditional support with rides, meals and special prayers.

# TABLE OF CONTENTS

# THE BEGINNING OF OUR JOURNEY

*The beginning of our story, yours and mine, starts with a strange dichotomy ... a strange contradiction between Life and the Olympics! Both have a starting line and both a finish line! For one, you eat and exercise and train and train to reach the finish line first; in case of the other, you have to eat and exercise and train and train, like an Olympian, each and every day, to reach the finish line last! And so, the title for this book, "PROSTATE CANCER The RACE to FINISH LAST!"*

In my case, with nearly a decade of encounter with PROSTATE CANCER and my previous writing experience, I was encouraged to write this book by my very competent and compassionate Oncologist, Dr. Daniel George (who heads up a team of prostate cancer specialist physicians, radiation oncologists, medical oncologists, physician assistants, research nurses, dieticians at The Duke Cancer Center in Durham, North Carolina, USA) to share my first-hand experience and to be of educational and emotional support for men, like me, facing prostate cancer.

Per the Center for Disease Control (CDC), 1 in 8 men or nearly <u>20 million</u> of us in the United States, who are likely to encounter prostate cancer during their lifetime, <u>I decided to write this book in terms as simple as possible, that can be easily understood, by those of us not associated with the field of medicine</u>.

Along my nearly decade long journey, I realized that besides the treatment itself, an understanding of supporting factors has made my journey more resolute and increased my endurance.

In the Chapters to follow, I have identified these supporting factors as Six (6) Pillars, that can be your guide in understanding <u>YOUR PROSTATE CANCER JOURNEY</u>!

# THE SIX (6) PILLARS

No cancer journey is easy, but can you, do it? YES, you can! If I have made it this far, so can you! The journey is all about 'attitude' and 'gratitude'! Along the way, I found that like me, a better understanding of these six supporting pillars will make your journey also more acceptable!

PILLAR 1 – UNDERSTANDING
THE PROSTATE

PILLAR 2 – PROSTATE CANCER –
DETECTION
AND TREATMENT

PILLAR 3 – THE MOST IMPORTANT
PERSON – YOU!

PILLAR 4 – YOUR SUPPORT SYSTEM–
FAMILY & FRIENDS

PILLAR 5 – MEDICAL INSURANCE

PILLAR 6 – PRAYER

# Chapter 1

*The beginning of our story, yours and mine, starts with a strange dichotomy ... a strange contradiction between Life and the Olympics! Both have a starting line and both a finish line! For one, you eat and exercise and train and train to reach the finish line first; in case of the other, you have to eat and exercise and train and train, like an Olympian, each and every day, to reach the finish line last! And so, the title for this book, "PROSTATE CANCER The RACE to FINISH LAST!"*

# Pillar 1

# Understanding the Prostate

**Pillar 1** – The first pillar on your prostate cancer journey is understanding the prostate.

**The Prostate** – The Prostate, an organ only in men, is a walnut-sized gland that surrounds the tube-shaped urethra, which runs from the bladder to the penis. Urine flows out of the bladder, through the urethra, to the penis.

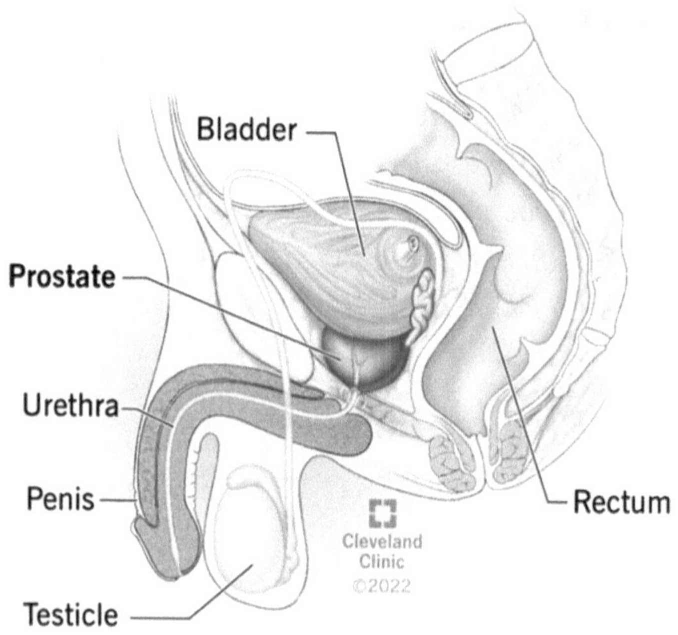

Bladder
Prostate
Urethra
Penis
Testicle
Rectum
Cleveland
Clinic
©2022

The primary purpose of the prostate is its significant role in a man's reproductive ability. During ejaculation, semen that is expelled, contains sperm produced by the testes (or testicles) and is combined with fluid secreted by the prostate, that nourishes and protects the sperm.

**Early Detection** - Most men ignore health-related issues until they get too advanced, when treatment and cure become more difficult. Early detection of any abnormality in the human body is helpful.

In case of the prostate, abnormalities can range from difficulty with starting urination; weak or interrupted flow of urine; urinating often, especially at night; trouble emptying the bladder completely; pain or burning during urination; or blood in the semen or urine. In my case, the prostate-related abnormality was blood in the semen.

**Prostate-related Issues** – If you are encountering one of the above abnormalities, a visit with your primary care physician can help identify whether your prostate-related issue is inflammation or swelling of the prostate (also referred to as Prostatitis), or an enlarged prostate, or in the worst case, prostate cancer. In my case, it turned out to be prostate cancer.

The condition of Prostatitis (inflammation or swelling of the prostate), is sometimes caused by infection and can be treated with antibiotics.

The condition of an Enlarged Prostate (also called BPH or Benign Prostate Hyperplasia) makes urination difficult, which may be controlled by using alpha-blockers to help relax the muscles around the urethra.

The condition of Prostate Cancer (the most common form of cancer in men besides skin cancer), according to the American Cancer Society, affects 1 in 8 men during their lifetime or roughly 20 million men in the United States. The most common forms of treatment can range from surgery to radiation to hormone therapy to chemotherapy.

**Testing by a Physician** – To understand your condition of the prostate, your primary care doctor will likely recommend a blood test to check your PSA level (Prostate-Specific Antigen) and perform a Digital Rectal Exam, with the word 'digital' coming from the Latin word 'digitus' meaning finger.

**Prostate-Specific Antigen (PSA)**: The prostate makes a protein called PSA or Prostate-Specific Antigen, which can be measured by a simple blood test. A high PSA may indicate an enlarged prostate or the possibility of prostate cancer. Within the medical community, opinions vary about the age at which a PSA blood test should be performed, but what is generally accepted is for men in their 60s, a PSA level above 4 ng/ml is considered abnormal.

**Digital Rectal Examination (DRE)**: As shown in Cleveland Clinic's sketch above, the prostate lies in front of the rectum, and a physician can feel the prostate by inserting a gloved, lubricated finger into the rectum. Because the physician checks the prostate through the rectum, some men mistakenly believe that the prostate is part of the gastrointestinal tract. In reality the prostate is part of a man's urinary system.

During a Digital Rectal Exam (DRE), a normal prostate feels relatively smooth.

A Digital Rectal Exam (DRE) that finds a smooth, soft prostate but which causes intense pain, is commonly a sign of infection, also known as Prostatitis and can be treated with antibiotics.

A Digital Rectal Exam (DRE) that finds a smooth, rubbery, and enlarged prostate is commonly a sign of prostate enlargement, also known as BPH or Benign Prostate Hyperplasia, and may be controlled by using alpha-blockers which help relax the muscles around the urethra.

A Digital Rectal Exam (DRE) that finds a hard nodule on the prostate may be a sign of prostate cancer and your primary care doctor will likely recommend you to see a UROLOGIST, a surgeon who treats diseases of the urinary system and the male reproductive system, which includes the prostate.

**Prostate Biopsy** – To rule out cancer, a sure way is to get tissue samples, referred to as a biopsy, and have the tissue samples diagnosed in a lab for the absence or presence of prostate cancer cells.

When having a surgical procedure, it is best to ask your surgeon and become aware of any side effects, you may encounter.

To perform the prostate biopsy, the Urologist will usually numb the area by injecting a local anesthetic, alongside the prostate and insert an ultrasound probe into the rectum. The ultrasound probe helps to guide the thin, hollow needle and remove a cylinder-shaped tissue from the prostate. The Urologist will repeat this procedure several times to get samples from different areas of the prostate.

In my case, the procedure was performed during an office visit and although it sounds painful, I only experienced brief discomfort, because the spring-loaded instrument inserts the thin, hollow needle and removes the tissue sample in a fraction of a second.

**Analysis of the Tissue Samples** – The tissue samples are sent to a Pathology lab, where they are sectioned, stained and read under a microscope by a Pathologist, a physician who reads and analyzes human tissue samples.

If the tissue samples show signs of cancer, which they did in my case, the next step is treatment.

**The Race to Finish Last!** - Now that you have an understanding of the first pillar, Understanding the Prostate, in the next chapter, Chapter 2 – (Pillar 2 - PROSTATE CANCER – DETECTION and TREATMENT), we'll cover how the severity of prostate cancer is measured and what my treatments have been over the past decade.

As you go through each pillar, do not lose sight of our objective, that you and I, are in this race to finish last! (the title of this book). No cancer journey is easy, but can you, do it? YES, you can! If I have made it this far, so can you!

**Alphabetic Refresher on Medical Terms:**

Digital Rectal Exam or DRE – feeling of the prostate by inserting a gloved, lubricated finger into the rectum

Enlarged Prostate - also called BPH or Benign Prostate Hyperplasia

Pathologist – a physician who reads and analyzes human tissue samples

Prostate – a walnut-sized organ only in men, that surrounds the tube-shaped urethra, which runs from the bladder to the penis

Prostate-Specific Antigen – also referred to as PSA

Prostatitis – inflammation or swelling of the prostate

Urethra – tube-shaped connector between the bladder and the penis

Urologist – a physician who treats diseases of the urinary system and the male reproductive system, including the prostate

# CHAPTER 2

*The beginning of our story, yours and mine, starts with a strange dichotomy ... a strange contradiction between Life and the Olympics! Both have a starting line and both a finish line! For one, you eat and exercise and train and train to reach the finish line first; in case of the other, you have to eat and exercise and train and train, like an Olympian, each and every day, to reach the finish line last! And so, the title of this book, "PROSTATE CANCER The RACE to FINISH LAST!"*

# PILLAR 2
# PROSTATE CANCER –
# DETECTION AND TREATMENT

**Pillar 2** – The second pillar on our prostate cancer journey is detection and treatment.

**Prostate Biopsy** – To rule out cancer, a sure way is to get tissue samples, referred to as a biopsy, and have the tissue samples diagnosed in a lab for the absence or presence of prostate cancer.

When having a surgical procedure, it is best to ask your surgeon and become aware of any side effects, you may encounter.

To perform the prostate biopsy, the Urologist will usually numb the area by injecting a local anesthetic alongside the prostate and insert an ultrasound probe into the rectum. The ultrasound probe helps to guide the thin, hollow needle and remove a cylinder-shaped tissue from the prostate. The Urologist will repeat this procedure several times to get samples from different areas of the prostate.

In my case, the procedure was performed during an office visit and although it sounds painful, I only experienced brief discomfort, because the spring-loaded instrument inserts the thin, hollow needle and removes the tissue sample in a fraction of a second.

**Analysis of the Tissue Samples** – The tissue samples are sent to a Pathology lab, where they are sectioned, stained and read under a microscope by a Pathologist (a physician who reads and analyzes human tissue samples), for the absence or presence of cancer.

Cancer cells may not show on every sample; but on the ones they do show, as they did in my case, the Pathologist will assign the cancer cells **a Gleason Scale grading from 1 to 5**, with Grade 1 if cancer looks a lot like normal prostate tissue, Grade 5 if cancer looks very abnormal and Grades 2 to 4 for features in between.

As explained by **The American Cancer Society**, the cancerous tissues often have areas with different grades. A grade is assigned to the two areas that make up most of the cancer. **These two grades are added up to give a Gleason Score (also called the Gleason Sum).**

Prostate cancers are divided into 3 groups -- low-grade if Gleason Score or Gleason Sum is 6 or less; intermediate-grade if Gleason Score or Gleason Sum is 7; and high-grade if Gleason Score or Gleason Sum is 8 to 10.

In my case, the Gleason Score or Gleason Sum was written as 4+5=9, which meant that most of my tumor was grade 4 and less was grade 5, for a total Gleason score of 9, which was very aggressive.

More aggressive the cancer, higher the risk of the cancer metastasizing, meaning prostate cancer cells spreading to other parts of the body, such as, lungs or bones. So, sooner prostate cancer is addressed, the better.

**Prostate Cancer Treatments** – Since there is no one cure for prostate cancer, Research Scientists and Drug Companies have been working on a variety of therapies and treatments. Depending on the severity level of the cancer, Prostate Cancer Oncologists around the country have applied a variety of treatments for their patients ranging from surgery, targeted radiation treatment, chemotherapy, immunotherapy, radioactive seed-implants, cryotherapy, hormone therapy (also called Androgen Deprivation Therapy or ADT), proton therapy, watchful waiting, clinical trials, metastasis-directed therapy which targets cancer-containing lymph nodes or bony areas with radiation and more therapies to come.

At first glance this range of treatments seems overwhelming, but to make you better informed, we'll discuss these treatments in more detail in Chapter 3 (Pillar 3 – The Most

Important Person – You!), so you can have a more educated and well-informed discussion with your Oncology team.

In the meantime, allow me to address what my prostate cancer journey has been over the past decade.

**My Prostate Cancer Journey** started after I first noticed blood in my semen. To rule out the possibility of infection, my primary care physician put me on two weeks of anti-biotics. When after two weeks of anti-biotics, I still noticed blood in the semen, my primary care physician referred me to a Urologist, who performed the biopsy of my prostate in his office.

A few days later, the Urologist called and informed me that the biopsy had shown cancer cells with a Gleason Score of 9 out of 10. The high Gleason Score meant a high risk for the prostate cancer to metastasize (meaning prostate cancer cells spreading to other parts of the body, such as lungs or bone).

Due to the aggressive nature of my prostate cancer, surgery to remove the prostate was recommended. After reviewing pros and cons of the surgery, pros being stopping metastasis (spreading of cancer cells to other parts of the body), cons being the possibility of temporary or permanent erectile dysfunction, I, along with my family, opted to have the prostate surgically removed.

The surgery called **Prostatectomy**, was performed with the surgeon using a De Vinci Robotics machine.

After removal of the prostate, I underwent 36 radiation sessions to radiate the prostate bed and reduce the chance of metastasis (of prostate cancer cells moving to other parts of the body).

For the next two years, my PSA was negligible and I was feeling fine. Then my PSA started to rise and a CT-Scan (Computed Tomography Scan) showed minor nodules in the lung. At this point, I opted for Dr. Daniel George at Duke Cancer Center in Durham, North Carolina to be my Oncologist, a very competent and compassionate physician.

Dr. Daniel George heads the Genitourinary (GU) Clinic and specializes in Urologic Cancers which include Prostate Cancer, Bladder Cancer, Kidney Cancer and Testicular Cancer. His very capable Oncology team includes surgeons, radiation oncologists, medical oncologists, physician assistants, research nurses and dieticians. Dr. George is also recipient of the Eleanor Easley Distinguished Professor Award in the School of Medicine, Medical Oncology.

I consider myself fortunate to be under his care.

Since the cancer had spread to the lungs, I had a more advanced PET Scan (Positron Emission Tomography), which is performed after injecting a safe FDA (Food and Drug Administration) approved radioactive tracer into the body. The tracer drug attaches to cancer cells, which "light up" on the screen.

My PET Scan showed an increase in the size of pulmonary (or lung) nodules and I was started on a regimen of Lupron injection every 6 months. **Lupron** is a hormone therapy to slow the production of male hormones (testosterone), which plays a role in the growth of prostate cancer cells.

At the same time, I was started on chemotherapy with a drug called **Docetaxel**, made from the bark of the rare Pacific yew tree. Injected by IV (intravenous), I received the Docetaxel chemotherapy in 6 sessions over a period of 17 weeks. To help fight the risk of infection during chemotherapy, a drug called **Neulasta**, was added in each session. Neulasta works by helping the body make white blood cells, which can reduce the risk of infection during chemotherapy.

For the next two years, after overcoming side effects of the chemo treatment (which in my case was mainly fatigue and hair loss), my lung nodules were stable and my PSA was undetectable.

After this time, when my PSA started rising again and CAT Scan showed a slight increase in the size of lung nodules, Dr. George started me on a daily oral Androgen Deprivation Therapy (ADT) medication called **Xtandi** (trade name for the medical term enzalutamide).

Androgen Deprivation Therapy (ADT) is a treatment to suppress or block production of male hormones (testosterone) which play a role in the growth of prostate cancer cells. Effects of ADT may include erectile dysfunction, low levels of testosterone, diminished energy.

A year later when my PSA started to increase and CT-Scan showed increase in size of lung nodules, I was started on an immunotherapy drug called **Provenge,** with 3 treatments over a course of 5 weeks. Immunotherapy drugs are designed to help our own immune system to kill cancer cells.

Our blood is made of white blood cells, red blood cells, plasma and platelets. In Provenge treatment, a process called leukapheresis is used, to remove white blood cells from your blood. Blood from your bloodstream is taken to separate white blood cells from the red blood cells, plasma and platelets.

The separated white blood cells are sent to a special lab to be processed with a genetically modified virus, returned about 3 days later and re-infused back into you intravenously.

Several months later, as my PSA was rising and lung nodules were growing, I was started on **Pluvicto**, a radio-nuclear targeted therapy. It is a radiation drug that targets cancer cells with the PSMA (Prostate Specific Membrane Antigen) marker, a protein found on most prostate cancer cells. After being injected into the body intravenously, radiation is released to damage and kill cancer cells.

Pluvicto (made from a rare earth element called Lutetium) has worked well for other prostate cancer patients; however, in my case after 3 treatments, when nodules continued to grow, it was decided to dis-continue treatment with Pluvicto.

I was then asked if I would be willing to participate in a trial with **PT-112**, a platinum-based therapy, which was in process of approval with the FDA (Food and Drug Administration). I agreed to participate and PT-112 was administered in 3 separate sessions over 6 weeks. Results for me were not favorable and decision was made to dis-continue the PT-112 therapy.

I next agreed to the **CHAMP trial** at Duke Cancer Center, consisting of two chemo drugs (Cabazitaxel and Carboplatin) and 2 immunotherapy drugs (Yervoy and Opdivo) to be administered every 3 weeks for up to 10 cycles. Medical term for Yervoy is ipilimumab and for Opdivo is nivolumab.

After the first infusion, due to stomach-related side effects, Yervoy was discontinued. I am now halfway through the study and so far, results have been good with cancer nodules being contained.

Even though some of the therapies have not worked well for me, it does not mean they would not work well for you.

**The Race to Finish Last!** - Now that you have an understanding of the first two pillars, in the next chapter, Chapter 3 – (Pillar 3 – THE MOST IMPORTANT PERSON – YOU!), we'll cover the variety of available therapies and treatments, so you can have a more educated and well-informed discussion with your Oncology team.

As you go through each pillar, do not lose sight of our objective, that you and I, are in this race to finish last! (the title of this book). No cancer journey is easy, but can you, do it? YES, you can! If I have made it this far, so can you!

**Alphabetic Refresher on Medical Terms:**

Androgen Deprivation Therapy (ADT) - a treatment to suppress or block production of male hormones (testosterone) which play a role in the growth of prostate cancer cells

Cabazitaxel – a chemotherapy drug

Carboplatin - a chemotherapy drug

CT-Scan - Computed Tomography Scan

Docetaxel – a chemotherapy drug made from the bark of the rare Pacific yew tree

FDA - Food and Drug Administration

Genitourinary (GU) – medical field that specializes in urologic cancers which include prostate cancer, bladder cancer, kidney cancer and testicular cancer

Gleason Scale – a numbering scale to identify severity of prostate cancer cells from 1 to 5, with grade 1 if cancer looks a lot like normal prostate tissue, grade 5 if cancer looks very abnormal and grades 2 to 4 for features in between

Gleason Score or Gleason Sum – addition of the Gleason number of two areas that make up most of the cancer in the biopsied prostate tissues

Immunotherapy – treatment that uses the body's own immune system to fight cancer

Leukapheresis – procedure where blood is taken from your bloodstream to separate white blood cells from the red blood cells, plasma and platelets

Lupron – a hormone therapy to slow the production of male hormones (testosterone), which plays a role in the growth of prostate cancer cells

Neulasta – a drug to help the body make white blood cells, which can reduce the risk of infection during chemotherapy

Opdivo – immunotherapy drug, for which medical term is nivolumab

PET Scan – Positron Emission Tomography Scan

PT-112 – a platinum-based therapy

Pluvicto - A radio-nuclear targeted drug, made from a rare earth element called Lutetium, to target cancer cells with the PSMA (Prostate Specific Membrane Antigen) marker, a protein found on most prostate cancer cells

Pathologist – a physician who reads and analyzes human tissue samples

Prostatectomy – surgery to remove the prostate

Provenge – an immunotherapy drug

PSMA – Prostate Specific Membrane Antigen

Yervoy – immunotherapy drug, for which medical term is ipilimumab

Xtandi – drug for which medical term is enzalutamide

# Chapter 3

*The beginning of our story, yours and mine, starts with a strange dichotomy ... a strange contradiction between Life and the Olympics! Both have a starting line and both a finish line! For one, you eat and exercise and train and train to reach the finish line first; in case of the other, you have to eat and exercise and train and train, like an Olympian, each and every day, to reach the finish line last! And so, the title of this book, "PROSTATE CANCER The RACE to FINISH LAST!"*

# Pillar 3
# The Most Important Person – You

**Pillar 3** – The third pillar on your prostate cancer journey is understanding that "you" are the most important person on this journey. The better equipped you are with knowledge of treatments and sources available and maintaining your emotional, mental and physical health, the more energized you will feel to navigate your prostate cancer journey!

In the previous chapter, I outlined my prostate cancer journey over the past decade, which starting with prostatectomy, has included radiation, chemotherapy, Lupron shots every 6 months, oral Xtandi pills, Provenge, Pluvicto, PT-112 and now the CHAMP trial with two chemo drugs Cabazitaxel + Carboplatin and immunotherapy drug Opdivo.

In this chapter, the most important person is YOU and the Prostate Cancer Journey you are going through with the three most important paths of your journey: 1) Keeping yourself informed of the variety of treatments available, 2) Maintaining your emotional and mental focus, and 3) Maintaining your physical health.

## 1.  KEEPING INFORMED on VARIETY of TREATMENTS AVAILABLE:

**Available Treatments** – Since there is no one cure for prostate cancer, Research Scientists and Drug Companies have been working on a variety of therapies and treatments. Depending on the severity level of the cancer, Prostate Cancer Oncologists around the country have applied a variety of treatments for their patients ranging from surgery, targeted radiation treatment, chemotherapy, immunotherapy, radioactive seed-implants, cryotherapy, hormone therapy (also called Androgen Deprivation Therapy or ADT), proton therapy, watchful waiting, clinical trials, metastasis-directed therapy which targets cancer-containing lymph nodes or bony areas with radiation and more therapies to come.

At first glance this range of treatments may seem overwhelming, but to make you better informed, let's discuss each one.

Surgery – referred to as Prostatectomy, is surgical removal of the prostate gland.

Radiation therapy – radiation to kill prostate cancer cells while minimizing damage to healthy cells.

Targeted Radiation Treatment – a non-invasive method of delivering radiation to the tumor that uses shaped beams to direct radiation at the cancer.

Chemotherapy – treatment that uses drugs to kill or stop the growth of cancer cells.

Immunotherapy – therapy that uses substances to stimulate our own immune system to help our body fight cancer.

Radioactive seed-implants – instead of radiation pointed at the prostate from outside the body, radioactive seeds are implanted into the prostate to kill cancer cells.

Cryotherapy – involves killing prostate cancer cells by freezing them.

Hormone therapy – also called Androgen Deprivation Therapy or ADT.

Proton Therapy – is a type of external beam therapeutic radiation. A beam of charged proton particles is generated by a large machine called a cyclotron and aimed at the prostate tumor. As the beam "deposits" its energy, it destroys the tumor cells.

Watchful Waiting – since prostate cancer is often slow growing, some men and their doctors may hold off on treatment and wait to see if the cancer appears to be growing.

Clinical Trials – through prostate cancer trials, researchers test the effects of new medications on a group of volunteers with prostate cancer.

Metastasis-directed Therapy – which targets cancer-containing lymph nodes or bony areas with radiation.

Focal Laser Ablation – use of extreme heat or cold on bone tumors to help ablate (destroy) them.


**Keeping Informed of developments through the non-profit Prostate Cancer Foundation**:

The Prostate Cancer Foundation (PCF.org or 1-800-757-CURE (2873) based in Santa Monica, California provides guides, such as 1) Patient Guide to Localized Prostate Cancer, 2) Patient Guide to Recurrent and Metastatic Prostate Cancer, 3) Additional Facts for Black Men, who have a higher risk of prostate cancer. The Foundation may also be able to find or recommend oncologists, who specialize in prostate cancer, in your geographic area.

**Keeping Informed of prostate cancer developments through trustworthy websites of Cancer Societies and Institutions around the country:**

American Cancer Society (cancer.org)

National Cancer Institute (cancer.gov)

American Society of Clinical Oncology (cancer.net)

**Keeping Informed on well-recognized Clinical Centers for treatment of Prostate Cancer around the country:** (per urologytimes.com)

Duke Cancer Center – Durham,
North Carolina

Cedars-Sinai Medical Center – Los Angeles,
California

Cleveland Clinic – Cleveland, Ohio

Johns Hopkins Medical Institutions –
Baltimore, Maryland

Mayo Clinic - Rochester, Minnesota

Mayo Clinic – Jacksonville, Florida

Mayo Clinic – Phoenix/Scottsdale, Arizona

Memorial Sloan – Kettering Cancer Center –
New York, New York

Loyola University Medical Center –
Chicago, Illinois

University of California Medical Center – San
Francisco, California

University of Iowa Holden Comprehensive
Cancer Center – Iowa City, Iowa

University of Kansas Medical Center –
Kansas City, Kansas

University of Texas M. D. Anderson Cancer
Center – Houston, Texas

Vanderbilt University Medical Center –
Nashville, Tennessee

Washington University Medical Center – St.
Louis, Missouri

If you live in the vicinity of and are able to
become a patient at one of these institutions, the

advantage (per Bottom Line Personal) may be having access to the very latest prostate cancer treatments, by signing up for clinical trials of a so-new-its-not-fully proven treatment or drug. In my case, I signed up for clinical trials at Duke Cancer Center in Durham, North Carolina and got treated with drugs such as Provenge, Pluvicto, PT-112 and Opdivo, which have been beneficial in prolonging my prostate cancer journey.

**Keeping Informed on Imaging Technologies** – Your Oncology team may use a variety of Advanced Imaging Technologies during your treatment, such as Magnetic Resonance Imaging (MRI), Computed Tomography (CT-Scan), or Positron Emission Tomography (PET Scan).

Magnetic Resonance Imaging (MRI) uses radio waves and strong magnets to create detailed images of soft tissues, such as tumors, in the body. A contrast agent, such as gadolinium, may be injected into the vein before the scan to better see details and determine the extent of the cancer. MRI can also show if cancer has spread outside of the prostate, which can be very important in determining your treatment options.

Computed Tomography (CT scan) scanners use a rotating X-ray tube and are normally done with and without contrast media, to improve the radiologist's ability to view the images inside the body. A contrast agent, such as dilute iodinated contrast may be injected into the vein before the scan.

Positron Emission Tomography (PET scan) can detect early changes in a patient's cells. CT scans and MRI show images of the patient's body organs, tissues and bones. PET scans, on the other hand, show how the patient's cells react to a special dye containing radioactive tracers, which may indicate cancerous areas.

Whereas CT scans and MRI can only detect changes later, PET scans can detect early changes in a patient's cells. Cancer cells have a higher level of chemical activity and often show up as bright spots on PET scans.

For prostate cancer patients, the new Prostate-Specific Membrane Antigen (PSMA) PET scan significantly improves how prostate cancer is detected and treated. The radioactive agent used binds to prostate cancer cells and is more effective in localizing metastatic prostate cancer.

## 2. MAINTAINING YOUR EMOTIONAL and MENTAL FOCUS:

**Be your own advocate** – be proactive and according to news caster John Roberts "never be afraid to ask questions" when it comes to your health!

**Your Oncology team** – if your Oncologist tells you, you have prostate cancer, ask for the Gleason Score. Based on how high your Gleason Score is, decide on the type of treatment. Develop a rapport with your Oncologist and his/her team. And, along your prostate cancer journey, keep a log of the activities associated with your treatments, such as infusions, drugs, diagnostic tests and so on. I have found keeping a log of treatments I have undergone, during my nearly decade long journey, to be helpful.

**Family and Friends support** – We will cover this in more detail in Chapter 4 (Pillar 4 – Your

Support System - Family and Friends), but appreciate your Caregiver, who can be the single rose in your garden, whether it is a family member or friend. As hard as the cancer journey is for you, it is as hard on your caregiver. Do not take them for granted and thank them often. For me, my wife has filled that role and I could not have come this far without her support.

**Insurance/Finance** – We will cover this in more detail in Chapter 5 (Pillar 5 – Medical Insurance).

**Prayer** – Prayer has helped me. If you feel prayer will help you, read Chapter 6 (Pillar 6 – Prayer). If you do not feel prayer helps, still read Chapter 6 for you may find it interesting!

**2-minute Meditation** – To help you relax a little, try meditation. Of all the books written on this subject, meditation is simply, sitting comfortably, closing your eyes and listening to yourself breath in and breath out.

**Joining a Prostate Cancer Support Group** – Google prostate cancer support group in my area, or google prostate cancer support group online.

So, let you and I, and our 20 million companions on our Prostate Cancer Journey, not become a statistic, for we all have a story! Everyone has a story … write how you are dealing with your journey to share and inspire others dealing with theirs.

## 3.  MAINTAINING YOUR PHYSICAL HEALTH:

**Mouth hygiene** – good health begins with a healthy mouth. Flossing minimizes food bacteria and helps make our gums healthier. So, brush and floss regularly.

**Water** – like plants, our human body needs sufficient water to keep our organs healthy. Start with a glass of water in the morning and stay sufficiently hydrated as advised by your doctor.

**Medication list** – keep your medication list (with name of drug, dosage level and number of pills a day) handy. For my convenience, I also keep my pills in a 2-week pill box, available at any pharmacy.

**Physical Pain** – If you experience physical pain, address it as early as possible. Unlike emotional or mental issues, physical pain cannot be shared with anyone else, so the earlier you address it the better.

**Move and Exercise** - Sitting is considered the new smoking! As a minimum, while watching TV and based on your physical agility, stand and sit during commercial breaks.

**Nutrition and Diet** – Dr. Peter Glidden has given a fine description of avoiding foods that hurt your body. "If you put diesel in an unleaded engine, it's going to run like crap, if it runs at all; nothing wrong with the car, just the wrong fuel". Same with the human body. Give it the right fuel and it will run better. Eat an anti-inflammatory diet low in animal products and processed foods and high in brightly-colored vegetables, whole grains, and beans.

**The Race to Finish Last!** – With an understanding of the first three pillars, in the next chapter, Chapter 4 (Pillar 4 – Your Support System - Family and Friends), we'll look at the importance of family and friends to make your prostate cancer journey as acceptable as possible.

As you go through each pillar, do not lose sight of our objective, that you and I, are in this race to finish last! (the title of this book). No cancer journey is easy, but can you, do it? YES, you can! If I have made it this far, so can you!

# CHAPTER 4

*The beginning of our story, yours and mine, starts with a strange dichotomy ... a strange contradiction between Life and the Olympics! Both have a starting line and both a finish line! For one, you eat and exercise and train and train to reach the finish line first; in case of the other, you have to eat and exercise and train and train, like an Olympian, each and every day, to reach the finish line last! And so, the title of this book, "PROSTATE CANCER The RACE to FINISH LAST!"*

# PILLAR 4
# YOUR SUPPORT SYSTEM –
# FAMILY AND FRIENDS

**Pillar 4** – The fourth pillar on your prostate cancer journey is understanding the importance of family and friends, who make up your support system and especially your Caregiver, for it has been well said that "to **have** a friend, you have to **be** a friend!"

**Your Caregiver** – Appreciate your caregiver, who is the single rose in your garden, whether it is a family member or friend. As hard as the cancer journey is for you, it is as hard on your caregiver. Caregivers are trying to juggle their existing roles and take over new responsibilities. So, do not take them for granted and thank them often. My wife has filled that role for me and I could not have come this far without her support.

If you are alone, try not to be lonely; reach out to Family and Friends for support.

Friends are people in your life, who want you to be in theirs. Ones who love to see you smile and lift you up no matter what.

There are friends, there is family and there are friends that become family.

Family and Friends are your companions on Your Prostate Cancer Journey for your Emotional, Mental and Physical support.

**Support from Family and Friends can help in so many ways:**

**Help with food and meals**

**Help with household chores**

**Help with running errands**

**Providing transportation to medical appointments**

**Discussing your treatments**

**Praying together** – If you believe in the power of prayer, prayers from family and friends can be a morale booster. Prayer has helped me.

**Discussing your finances and insurance**

**Help with scanning websites**

**Sharing your outdoor hobbies** – such as fishing or carpentry

**Sharing with family and friends a new indoor hobby you may like to develop** – such as,

American Presidents (one of my favorite subjects)

Astronomy (Planets; Stars, Comets, Galaxies)

Astrology (12 signs of the Zodiac related to the elements of fire, earth, air, and water. Fire: Aires, Leo, Sagittarius. Earth: Taurus, Virgo,

Capricorn. Air: Gemini, Libra, Aquarius.
Water: Cancer, Scorpio, Pisces)

Mythology (Zeus, Apollo, Aphrodite, Athena, gods of Olympus)

Ornithology (Birds as Hummingbirds, Cardinals, other exotic species)

Geography (close to 200 Countries on seven Continents and five major Oceans)

Music (12 notes per octave, each with its unique pitch; wind instruments as flutes and trumpets versus stringed instruments as pianos and violins)

Wines (whites, as Chardonnay and Sauvignon Blanc; reds as Merlot and Cabernet Sauvignon; rose and dessert wines; sparkling like Champagne and Prosecco)

Gemology (Precious stones as Emeralds, Diamonds, Rubies)

Botany (Flowers as Daffodils, Roses, Lilies)

World Empires (as British, Roman, Ottoman)

Dynasties (as Egyptian, Chinese, Indian)

At the tip of your fingers, google your topic of interest, such as "basics of wines" or "basics of music" to find the resources to sharpen your mind, and inspire you to find your niche.

**The Race to Finish Last!** – As critical as understanding the first four pillars of your prostate cancer journey are, equally important is understanding your medical insurance and, if getting close to age 65, selecting the Medicare program that best fits your needs, as covered in the next chapter, Chapter 5 (Pillar 5 – Medical Insurance).

As you go through each pillar, do not lose sight of our objective, that you and I, are in this race to finish last! (the title of this book). No cancer journey is easy, but can you, do it? YES, you can! If I have made it this far, so can you!

# CHAPTER 5

*The beginning of our story, yours and mine, starts with a strange dichotomy ... a strange contradiction between Life and the Olympics! Both have a starting line and both a finish line! For one, you eat and exercise and train and train to reach the finish line first; in case of the other, you have to eat and exercise and train and train, like an Olympian, each and every day, to reach the finish line last! And so, the title of this book, "PROSTATE CANCER The RACE to FINISH LAST!"*

# PILLAR 5
# MEDICAL INSURANCE

**Pillar 5** – The fifth pillar on your prostate cancer journey is the understanding of coverage and cost of your medical insurance, whether it be Medicare or insurance through work or military-related insurance.

Most prostate cancer patients are approaching age 65 or are age 65 and older.

65 is the age when people become eligible for Medicare, a federal health insurance program for people age 65 and older and for younger people with certain disabilities.

**Original Medicare versus Medicare Advantage Programs** – Understanding and signing up for Medicare benefits can be confusing! According to aarp.org, it is not one size fits all. Depending on your personal situation, the key issue is deciding to go with Original Medicare or with a Medicare Advantage Plan. Your personal decision will be based on factors such as premiums, out-of-pocket costs and choice of doctors.

As explained by medicareinteractive.org, let us first understand the 4 parts of Medicare: Part A, Part B, Part C and Part D.

- Part A provides Inpatient/ Hospital coverage
- Part B provides Outpatient/ Medical coverage
- Part C offers an alternate way to receive your Medicare benefits (we'll discuss below)

–     Part D provides prescription
      drug coverage

Original Medicare, sometimes called Traditional Medicare, is made up of Medicare Part A + Part B. Original Medicare does not cover Part D (Prescription Drugs).

Some of the items and services not covered by Medicare include:

–     Long term care (also called
      custodial care)
–     Most dental care
–     Eye exams (for prescription glasses)
–     Dentures
–     Cosmetic surgery
–     Massage therapy
–     Routine physical exams
–     Hearing aids and exams for
      fitting them

Per medicare.gov, for **Part A** most people do not pay a premium. Part A covers inpatient care in a hospital, in a skilled nursing facility (that is not long-term care), lab tests, end-of-life hospice care.

For **Part B** you pay a premium which is deducted from your Social Security check each month. Part B helps cover services from doctors and other health care providers, outpatient care, home health care, durable medical equipment (like wheelchairs, walkers, hospital beds and other equipment).

After you meet your Part B deductible, Part B usually pays 80% of allowable charges for a covered service. After that, you are responsible for paying 20% of the Medicare-approved amount for your care.

The 20%, not paid by Original Medicare, can be a significant amount, for which you can purchase private insurance for a Medicare Supplement Policy (also referred to as Medigap). As an alternative, you can join a Medicare Advantage Plan (Part C) offered by private health insurance companies, for which we will discuss the pros and cons below.

**Part C** Medicare Advantage Plans combine coverage of Medicare Part A and Part B into a single plan and may provide additional benefits such as prescription drug coverage, dental coverage, vision, and hearing services.

**Part D** provides prescription drug coverage. Part D is provided only through private insurance companies that have contracts with the government and each plan covers a different list (or formulary) of drugs. If you want prescription drug coverage with Original Medicare, you have to choose and join a stand-alone Part D private drug plan (PDP).

**Pros and Cons of Original Medicare with a Supplement Policy versus a Medicare Advantage Plan** - It is important to understand your Medicare choices and pick your coverage carefully.

**Coverage:** Original Medicare covers Part A and Part B but does not cover Part D (Prescription Drugs). Medicare Advantage Plans cover Part A and Part B, and depending on the Advantage Plan you choose, may also cover items such as prescription drugs, routine visual exam and dental care.

**Doctors and Hospitals**: In Original Medicare, you are allowed to go directly to nearly all doctors and hospitals in the country, and rarely requires prior permission or authorization from Medicare or your primary care doctor. On the other hand, Medicare Advantage Plans, typically have network restrictions and may require prior authorization, meaning that you will likely be more limited in your choice of doctors and hospitals.

**Premiums and Out-of-Pocket Costs**: Premiums and out-of-pocket costs vary between purchasing insurance for Medigap Supplement Policies (if you decide to go with Original Medicare) versus premiums and out-of-pocket costs, such as deductibles for a Medicare Advantage Plan you choose. Note: Medigap Supplement Policies go by letters, such as C, D, G and depending on the plan you choose, it may cover all or part of the 20% you are responsible for.

There are a number of government programs that may help reduce your health care and prescription drug costs, if you meet the eligibility requirements.

Some websites about Medicare that can be helpful are medicare.gov, aarp.org, medicareinteractive.org

**The Race to Finish Last!** - The first five pillars embody the physical part of the prostate cancer journey. The next chapter, Chapter 6 (Pillar 6 – Prayer) is optional. Prayer has helped me. If you feel prayer will help you, read on. If you do not feel prayer helps, still read Chapter 6, for you may find it interesting!

As you go through each pillar, do not lose sight of our objective, that you and I, are in this race to finish last! (the title of this book). No cancer journey is easy, but can you, do it? YES, you can! If I have made it this far, so can you!

**Alphabetic Refresher of Terms:**

AARP – American Association of Retired Persons

Hospice Care – end-of-life care

Long-term Care – also called custodial care

Original Medicare - Part A + Part B and does not cover Part D (prescription drugs)

# Chapter 6

*The beginning of our story, yours and mine, starts with a strange dichotomy ... a strange contradiction between Life and the Olympics! Both have a starting line and both a finish line! For one, you eat and exercise and train and train to reach the finish line first; in case of the other, you have to eat and exercise and train and train, like an Olympian, each and every day, to reach the finish line last! And so, the title of this book, "PROSTATE CANCER The RACE to FINISH LAST!"*

# Pillar 6
# Prayer

**Pillar 6** – The sixth pillar on your prostate cancer journey, if it inspires you, is prayer. For thousands of years before the I-phone, the earliest form of wireless communication was prayer!

If prayer inspires you, read on ... ... for regardless of faith or religion, I have found prayer, not only my prayers, but prayers from family and friends, to uplift me on my prostate cancer journey.

If you accept organized religion as your form of worship, you may be interested in the evolution of world religions, for all major religions of the world started on the continent of ASIA.

## Middle East

| Religion | Founder | Place |
| --- | --- | --- |
| Zoroastrian | Zoroaster | Persia |
| Judaism | Abraham | Babylon |
| Christianity | Christ | Jerusalem |
| Islam | Muhammad | Mecca |

## From East Asia

| Religion | Founder | Place |
| --- | --- | --- |
| Hinduism | The Brahmins | India |
| Buddhism | Buddha | India |
| Jainism | Mahavira | India |
| Sikhism | Guru Nanak | India |
| Taoism | Laozi | China |
| Shinto | not known | Japan |

The three monotheistic religions of Judaism, Christianity, and Islam came from the House of Abraham with Isaac born from wife Sarah, and Ishmael from Hagar.

From the lineage of Isaac came Jews and Christians and from the lineage of Ishmael came Muslims.

Jews revere Yahweh; Christians revere Christ; Muslims revere Allah.

Jews follow the Torah; Christians follow the Bible; Muslims follow the Koran.

The three main groups of Christianity are The Roman Catholic Church, Protestant Churches (as Anglican, Lutheran, Episcopalian, Presbyterian, Methodist, Baptist, and more), and The Orthodox Church (as Russian, Syrian, Ethiopian, and more).

The two sects of Islam, Sunni and Shia originated from a power struggle for succession, immediately following the passing of Prophet Muhammad. Sunnis (followers of then-ruling class of Caliphas), and Shias (followers of the descendants of Prophet Muhammad). The assassination of Prophet Muhammad's grandsons Hassan and Hussein generated the Sunni-Shia conflict that has been on-going for the past 1,400 years. Today, this conflict continues between Sunni Saudi Arabia and Shiite Iran, as to who is the rightful custodian of Islam; Saudi Arabia, guardian of Mecca, the holiest site of Islam, or Iran, the Shiite followers of the descendants of Prophet Muhammad.

It should also be noted that most Christians are unaware of Islam's reverence to Mary (mother of Christ) in the Koran. Considered the holiest of women, she is the only woman referred by name in the Koran and the entire chapter 19 is devoted to Mary in the Koran. Christ, not considered son of God, but is considered the second highest Prophet after Prophet Muhammad.

To know more about a religion, google "basic belief of (name of religion)".

**The Race to Finish Last!** As you go through each pillar, do not lose sight of our objective, that you and I, are in this race to finish last! (the title of this book). No cancer journey is easy, but can you, do it? YES, you can! If I have made it this far, so can you!

# PROSTATE CANCER
# THE RACE
# TO
# FINISH LAST!

## RAFIQ BANDUKWALA

TO MY 20 MILLION FELLOW
COMPANIONS ON OUR JOUNEY.
THANK YOU FOR READING THE BOOK
AND HOPE IT WILL BRIGHTEN UP <u>YOUR</u>
<u>PROSTATE CANCER JOURNEY!</u>

# ABOUT THE AUTHOR

RAFIQ BANDUKWALA, (author of book titled DON'T RE'TIRE', RE'FRESH'! A Refreshing Look at Retirement available on Amazon), is a graduate of St. Xavier's High School, Mumbai, India, of College of Engineering, Pune, India and received his post graduate engineering degree from North Carolina State University in Raleigh, North Carolina.

With nearly a decade of my encounter with PROSTATE CANCER and my previous writing experience, I was encouraged to write this book by my brilliant and compassionate Oncologist, Dr. Daniel George of Duke Cancer Center in Durham, North Carolina, USA, who heads up a team of Prostate Cancer specialist Physicians, Physician Assistants, Research Nurses and Nutritional Dieticians.

With nearly 20 million of my fellow companions in the United States who are likely to encounter Prostate Cancer during their lifetime, I decided to write this book in terms as simple as possible that can be easily understood by those of us not associated with the field of medicine.

And finally, as in my case, I identify the Six Pillars in six different chapters to be your guide in understanding <u>YOUR PROSTATE CANCER JOURNEY</u>!

www.ingramcontent.com/pod-product-compliance
Lightning Source LLC
Chambersburg PA
CBHW031424250726

48656CB00002B/814